Robert Wadlow

The Unique Life of the Boy
Who Became the World's Tallest Man

by Jennifer Phillips

ISBN 1453829474   EAN13 9781453829479

Cover image: Robert posing with his mother in February 1939, a little more than a year before he died. Images on the cover and pages 8, 12, 16, 19, 20, 24, 29 and 33 are courtesy of *The Telegraph* newspaper in Alton, Illinois.

"The most outstanding thing about him was that he had such a pleasant smile. I really can't recall seeing Robert without this pleasant smile on his face."

Classmate Ruby Harris

Imagine You Are a Giant. You tower over your school friends and even grown-ups. You need special clothes and shoes. Your feet are too long for most stairs. Furniture is too small. People stare. Sometimes, they even pinch or kick your legs to see if you are using stilts.

Meanwhile, your body just keeps growing and growing with no end in sight. You are a giant, but your size doesn't come with superhuman strength or spine-tingling excitement. Just getting through your day takes a lot of energy.

How would you feel?

This was Robert Wadlow's experience.

He probably had days when he felt scared, frustrated, embarrassed or uncomfortable. Yet he was known for being patient, gentle, smart and funny. His size came with hardships, but he learned how to cope.

He refused to be angry about the different life he had to lead.

Robert, you see, became the world's tallest man. He stood almost nine feet tall by the time of his death.

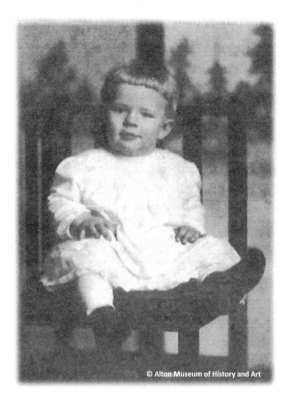

Robert at six months old.

Just a Growth Spurt? February 22, 1918, began as a frosty winter morning when Addie Wadlow gave birth to Robert in the five-room cottage she shared with her husband, Harold. They lived in Alton, Illinois, a small Midwestern town perched along the Mississippi River.

Robert was a regular-sized 8½-pound baby. The first months of his life showed no signs of the unusual journey to follow.

Even when Robert started sprouting up fast as a toddler, his parents didn't worry too much. They had their hands full as first-time parents. They figured their son was just having an early growth spurt.

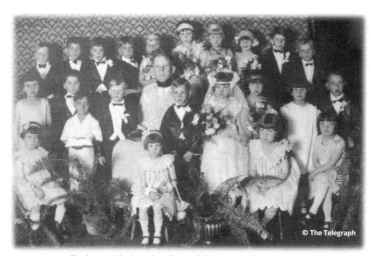

*Robert, sitting in the middle row fourth from the left,
as a third grader in the school play.*

A Boy in a Man's Body. But the growth spurt didn't stop. Soon, Robert's size could no longer be overlooked.

By age five, Robert was adult size. This confused people. Train and bus drivers wanted to charge him regular ticket prices. People forgot his young age and expected him to talk like a grown-up.

Robert took little notice. His friends didn't seem to care, either. To them, he was just Bob, a curious and happy neighborhood boy who enjoyed things like baseball, marbles, sledding, swimming, watching western movies and using his imagination to make up games.

People really got talking when Robert was ready to start school. They fretted and wondered about how Robert would fit in. Not

Robert. For him, school was an exciting new world he joined eagerly. He quickly earned the affection of his teachers and classmates.

During these early years, the Wadlow family moved back and forth between Illinois, West Virginia and Colorado. They settled back in Alton for good when Robert started the third grade.

By this point, Robert stood about six feet, taller than many American adults. His carefree years of ignoring his size ended. He continued to grow and the classroom became uncomfortable.

His weight could break a regular chair. His legs barely fit under a school desk. He had trouble holding pencils and other school supplies with his large hands. Blackboards, doors, bulletin boards and drinking fountains loomed painfully low. His ears rang with the constant *gong!* of school bells perched high out of the way for everyone but him. Robert's clumsy movements also made little accidents common.

The school did what it could to make things bearable. His classmates and teachers really liked Robert. With his shy smile, quiet intelligence and nose constantly in a book, he didn't expect to be treated differently.

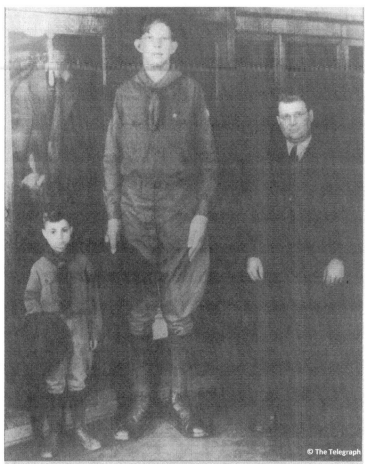

Robert P. Wadlow became the world's tallest Boy Scout when he was 13 years old. He was 7 feet 4 inches tall and his uniform was specially made. Here Robert models his new uniform, ordered by Alton clothier Carl Hartmann. Another Boy Scout wears the regular-size uniform. Telegraph archive photo.

Newspaper clipping of Robert showing off his Boy Scout uniform.

The World Discovers Robert. Life changed when Robert was nine. Newspaper reporters learned of his unusual size. Before long, he was known around the world.

People flocked to Alton to see the "giant boy" themselves. Some behaved respectfully, some did not. Circuses still recruited people with deformities to be in freak shows at this time. Offers came in for Robert to go on display because of his remarkable height. His family wanted nothing to do with this.

"As far as circuses are concerned, I wouldn't join one if it was the last thing on earth," Robert said. "There are too many people who stretch their necks at me now."

Robert never experienced true privacy again.

At first, the publicity embarrassed and bothered him. He wanted to be left alone and do normal things like a normal boy. Luckily, his family and school friends were very caring. They helped to protect him from outsiders.

By the time Robert was fourteen, the Wadlow family included sisters Helen and Betty along with brothers Eugene and Harold Jr. Robert treasured being with family. He loved discussing new ideas with his dad. He played hide and seek with his youngest brother, Harold. And he enjoyed hanging out at his aunt's nearby farm, where he savored treats such as fresh peaches and cream or warm homemade bread slathered with butter.

His family surrounded him with love and normal moments in their simple home. This helped Robert endure the outside attention. He discovered a new level of patience.

"I have got used to being stared at," he later told a newspaper reporter. "To resent it would only make folks unhappy, including myself. Some people say unkind things, of course. I thought it over long ago and decided to ignore them. The worst you can say about them is that they are thoughtless."

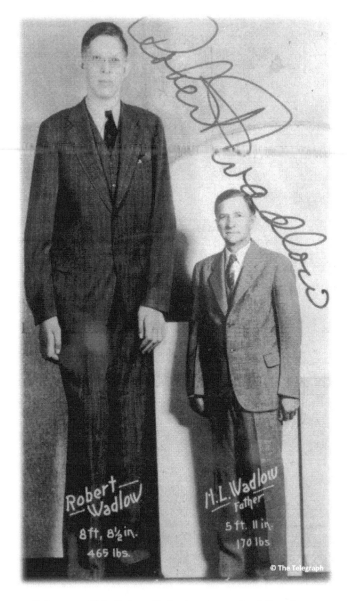

Robert and his father. Robert autographed the photo at someone's request.

A Medical Discovery. No one else in the Wadlow family was extra tall. Just before Robert turned twelve, doctors figured out why he was growing so fast and so large.

It involved his overactive pituitary gland. This small, egg-shaped organ near the back of the brain helps control people's growth. Robert's gland was making too much of a substance called a growth hormone.

This condition is now called gigantism and some people still suffer from it. But no one has grown as tall as Robert yet.

Doctors and Robert's family decided against a risky surgery to try and fix the problem. Still, doctors wanted to study Robert. They hoped to treat or even prevent such problems with other people in the future.

Robert had a good relationship with his doctors, but he went through many uncomfortable medical tests over the years. He didn't enjoy this at all but agreed to help with medical research.

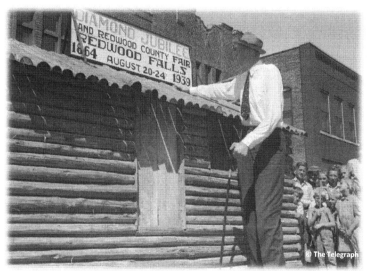

Robert on tour in Redwood Falls, Minnesota.

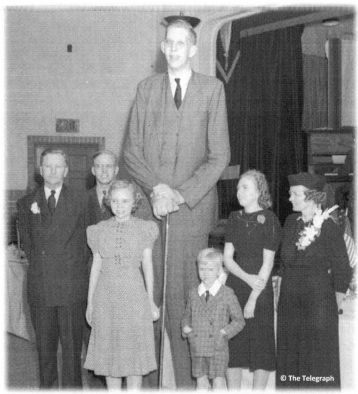

Robert with his family in 1939. From left: Harold Sr., Eugene, Betty, Harold Jr., Helen, Addie.

The Problem of Clothes. Robert did enjoy a good laugh. He had a healthy sense of humor.

He chuckled and blushed when gently teased by his friends. He played harmless jokes, such as taking someone's hat and hanging it out of reach on a chandelier. He smiled about handing down too-small clothes to his father or seeing them used as fabric for his younger sisters.

Robert's parents were glad their oldest son could handle his predicament so well, even as they worried about family expenses. It was tough enough raising a family in the 1920s and 1930s. Jobs were hard to find. Money and food were in short supply for many Americans.

As Robert kept springing up, he needed specially made clothes. His parents "sent my measurements in for a suit," Robert once told a reporter, "but the company kept sending them back saying they were a mistake."

Shoes were a big problem. Factories figured out a special way to make Robert's size, but the shoes often were too small when they arrived months later because Robert grew so fast. Eventually, his foot grew to more than nineteen inches long.

The family needed help making ends meet. Robert started appearing as a shoe company spokesman when he was twelve in exchange for his shoes. He began to like speaking in public. He even took a class to practice his skills.

"He naturally was very clumsy because he was so big. He would fall easily and always tear the knees out of his pants. His mother would take these pants to a dressmaker in Alton and have girls' skirts made out of the backs of the legs."

Cousin Mina Cornine

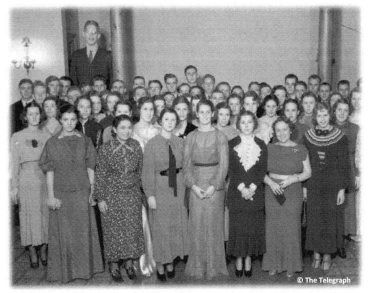

Robert with his Alton High School graduating class in 1936.

Finding His Place in the World.

Every birthday, reporters updated the world about Robert.

People were treated to new pictures of the sandy-haired youth with his pleasant smile, tinted round glasses and large ears poking out. Photographs always showed him dressed neatly in a formal suit or zip-up sweater with tie and slacks.

He received lots of cards and presents from strangers wishing him well. He especially liked gifts of books. He devoured hundreds of books every year and tried hobbies like stamp collecting, swimming, basketball and photography.

In the seventh grade, he nominated himself for student body president and won. He even became the world's tallest Boy Scout.

As a teenager, Robert began to accept his unusual life. His size was hard on his body and health. It even kept him out of high school for several weeks while he recovered from an illness that started with an infected toe.

But his size also gave him a stepping stone to interesting opportunities. He enjoyed traveling. He loved geography and history. Working for the shoe company took him to eight hundred towns in forty-one states. Mr. Wadlow traveled along with him to protect, encourage and just enjoy being with his son.

Travel wasn't comfortable. Robert had to squeeze into regular seats, beds, bathtubs and rooms. His family came up with inventive solutions. To travel by car, for example, his father removed the front passenger seat so Robert could stretch out from the back.

He liked meeting new people and seeing new places. With a special fondness for children, he always made an effort to visit schools, orphanages and children's hospitals.

People who met Robert were humbled by his gracious behavior.

"How's the weather up there?" people asked over and over, thinking the question was clever. He patiently smiled or replied, even though he didn't find it so clever.

He agreed to participate in a circus show only once. In 1937, when he was nineteen, he appeared in the Ringling Brothers and Barnum & Bailey Circus for a few weeks. Wearing his usual dress pants, shirt and tie, he stood in the center ring twice a day for a few minutes while an announcer introduced him.

Televisions were not common yet, so people listened to radio shows for news and entertainment. A radio interview broadcast during one of his New York visits gave Americans a rare chance to hear Robert's unusually deep voice, caused by his enlarged vocal chords.

Did Robert ever get frustrated about his situation? Yes! He didn't like people poking his legs to see if he was pretending. And he didn't like others complaining about their problems. He felt blessed. He wanted others to appreciate what life gave them.

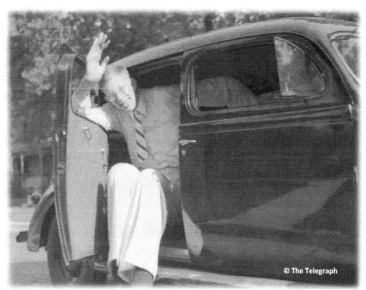

© The Telegraph

Robert leaving for a tour of the western United States.

The Unique Life of the Boy Who Became the World's Tallest Man

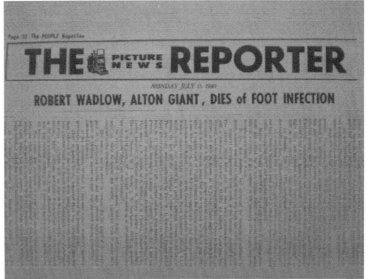

Robert's untimely death was news around the world.

An Early Death. Robert's body size began taking a dangerous toll on his health by the time he was a young man going to college.

He could only walk a short distance and he needed to use a cane. He started losing feeling below the knees. His feet could be injured easily. The icy Illinois winters threatened him with bone-breaking falls. He had trouble holding pens, pencils and science lab instruments needed in his college classes.

His dreams of becoming a lawyer started to fade.

Robert pondered his future and decided to change direction. He started traveling again for the shoe company. He wanted to save money and open his own shoe store or even a chain of stores.

Robert's plan seemed on track until a trip to Michigan with his father in 1940. Robert was twenty-two years old and towered over everyone at 8 feet 11.1 inches tall. He weighed 439 pounds. His giant size meant his body could not heal easily from injury or illness.

His ankle brace, worn to give his bones more support, caused a blister. This became infected. Robert turned very ill, fighting a fever that soared to 106 degrees. The infection spread throughout his body. Doctors tried for ten days to save Robert.

Early on the morning of July 15, 1940, he died in his sleep.

News of Robert's death spread quickly around the world. His family brought him back to Illinois for his burial. At least forty thousand people traveled to Alton to say good-bye in the days before his funeral service and about 10,000 attended the service. When the funeral began, the entire city paused for five minutes to silently honor their fallen son.

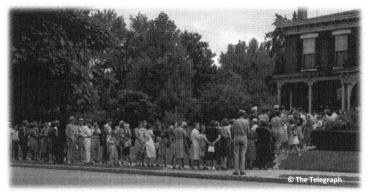

People wait in line outside the funeral home to file past Robert's casket.

Robert brought joy to his family and friends while inspiring millions of people with his courage and patience. He also helped scientists learn more about medical problems like his.

He will always be remembered for his fantastic size, but his gift to the world was much greater than his height.

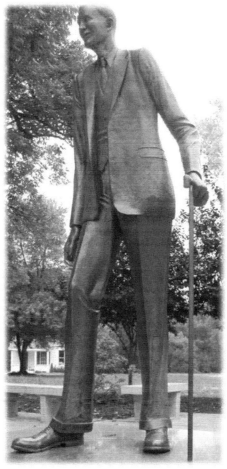

People from all over the world visit Robert's statue in upper Alton.
A life-size bronze replica of a chair he used sits nearby
for visitors to try.

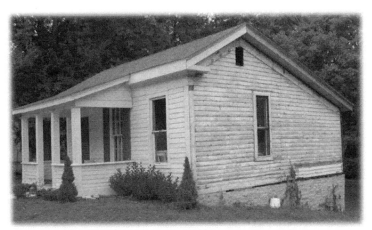

The Alton museum is working to restore the house
where Robert was born.

You can learn more about Robert Wadlow and order other materials through the Alton Museum of History & Art: www.altonmuseum.com.

More Facts to Note

Medicines that might have saved Robert's life weren't yet available. For example, the antibiotic penicillin became more widely distributed in 1943—three years after his death.

A handful of people are known to have grown past 8 feet tall. But Robert remains the only person with a verified height measurement of 8' 11.1". He still holds a place in the Guinness Book of World Records as the tallest man in history.

After Robert's death, his parents worried about curiosity seekers. They had his casket placed in a vault and the grave encased in concrete and steel. Many of his belongings were burned.

Harold Wadlow Sr. collaborated with one of Robert's college professors on a biography released the year after Robert's death. Mr. Wadlow then turned down other requests over the years to publish more books about his son.

All of Robert's immediate family— his parents, sisters and brothers—are buried alongside his grave in Alton, Illinois.

Timeline

February 22, 1918	Robert born
1920	Sister Helen born
1922	Brother Eugene born
1924	Sister Betty born
February 1927	The press first learns about Robert
January 1929	Over-active pituitary gland discovered as cause behind Robert's extraordinary growth
Summer 1930	Starts appearing on behalf of the Peters Shoe Company of St. Louis
1931	Joins Boy Scouts
1932	Brother Harold Jr. born
	Starts at Alton Senior High School
February 1935	Misses last semester of high school due to foot infection and influenza
January 24, 1936	Completes make-up semester, graduates with 86 other students from high school class
February 1936	Enrolls in Shurtleff College in Alton
Fall 1936	Decides to raise money and go into business instead of finishing college
July 15, 1940	Dies from infection while on trip to Michigan at age 22

Questions to Explore

❖ **People are different in many ways. Robert Wadlow stood out because he was extra tall compared to typical Americans**

> What are other ways a person can feel different? Can this change based on the region or country where you live?

❖ **Extra tall people sometimes hear remarks such as, "How's the weather up there?" These comments may sound more amusing than they really are.**

> What else might people say or ask others without thinking about how it feels?

❖ **When Robert was alive, circuses still featured people with unusual physical features and called them freaks. Many of these people lived very unhappy lives and were not treated like ordinary people.**

> How have attitudes changed? Are there some ways that times haven't changed?

❖ **Robert seemed to cope for the most part with his unusual size and constant attention.**

What do you think helped him the most?

❖ **Most people feel different in some way.**

What do you find different about yourself? If it bothers you or makes it harder for you to do something, what helps you cope?

Activities

❖ **Use an encyclopedia or education web site to learn about important events happening around the world while Robert was alive.**

Look up topics such as the Roaring 20s, Great Depression and the growing conflict that would become World War II soon after Robert's death.

❖ **Measure 8 feet 11.1 inches (or round up to 9 feet) on a floor or wall. Compare your height to Robert's when he was a young adult. (Or measure 6 feet to see his height in the third grade.)**

What else is this tall, deep or long?

❖ **Pretend to use a toothpick as a pencil to understand how awkward it became for Robert to write with his large hands.**

❖ **Find a too-small desk or chair to sit in for awhile (maybe preschool-size furniture).**

❖ Trace an outline of your foot on a large piece of paper. Then trace a larger foot outline around this shape. Make this shape measure 18 1/2 inches long, about 5 inches wide at the heel and almost 6 inches wide at the ball of the foot. This was Robert's shoe size when he was 12.

Make a paper cutout to use in helping others learn about Robert.

❖ Measure 96 inches. This was the length of Robert's shoelaces.

How long are your shoelaces?

❖ Research other extra-tall people from history. Try to find information on people such as Sandy Allen, Yao Defen, Leonid Stadnik, Bao Xishun and Alexander Sizonenko.

What is the tone of the coverage you find? Are their situations and lives handled with respect? How can you tell if information about their lives and heights seems accurate?

Bibliography

Primary Sources

Alton Telegraph. Various newspaper articles about Robert Wadlow's life and interviews with the Wadlow family. Hayner Library's Illinois Room Collection, Alton, Illinois: www.haynerlibrary.org.

Robert Wadlow Collection. Archival information and artifacts. Alton Museum of History and Art, Alton, Illinois: www.altonmuseum.com.

The Story of Robert, videotape including rare film footage and interviews, Valley Park, Missouri: CTL Productions, 1991.

Voices of the River Bend. CD with broadcast of 1937 New York radio interview given by Robert Wadlow, Alton Museum of History and Art, Alton, Illinois: www.altonmuseum.com.

Other Materials

Bottens, Mary Kay. *Stand Tall. A Story of Robert P. Wadlow,* Stand Tall Publishers, 1992.

Brannon, Dan. *Boy Giant. The Story of Robert Wadlow. The World's Tallest Man,* Alton, Illinois: Museum of History & Art, 2003.

Dimmer, Frederick, *Incredible People. Five Stories of Extraordinary Lives,* New York: Atheneum Books for Young Readers, 1997.

Dimmer, Frederick. *Very Special People. The Struggles, Loves and Triumphs of Human Oddities,* New York: Bell Publishing Co., 1985.

Fadner, Frederick. *The Gentleman Giant. The Biography of Robert Pershing Wadlow,* Mt. Vernon, Indiana: Windmill Publications, originally published 1941, reprinted 1998.

Landau, Elaine. *Standing Tall. Unusually Tall People,* New York: Franklin Watts, 1997.

Mooney, Julie. *The World of Ripley's Believe It Or Not!,* New York: Black Dog and Leventhal Publishers, 1999.

Acknowledgments

Finding reproduction-quality images to use in historical biographies can be a challenge. I owe my success directly to Charlotte ("Char") Stetson, archivist at *The Alton Telegraph*. She enthusiastically helped me out with images to include in this book.

The staff and volunteers at the Alton Museum of History and Art helped with numerous questions over the past several years. Staff in the Genealogy & Indexing Department at The Hayner Public Library in Alton provided a nice collection of photocopied newspaper articles for me to reference.

Writer/editor extraordinaire Carla Intlekofer provided invaluable editing support. And, last but not least, is my family (comprised of one husband, two daughters and one bird). They accept my writing (and poor knitting) as facts of life and support me with the precious gift of time for power naps to offset my early morning work habit.

About the Author

Jennifer Phillips grew up in Alton, Illinois and doesn't remember a time when she didn't know Robert Wadlow's story. There were school field trips to the Wadlow Room at the Franklin Masonic Lodge and visits to the Alton museum. Even now, she always visits Robert's statue when going home.

A former newspaper reporter, Jennifer lives in Shoreline, Washington and likes to write about almost anything and everything. She especially likes writing for children but has done her share of writing for grown-ups (mainly non-fiction and corporate information).

You can find a learning guide and short video trailer for use with this book (plus more children's writing) at her Web site, www.noseinabookpublishing.com. She has published two other biographies to date: *Elijah Lovejoy's Fight for Freedom* and *Nina Kosterina: A Young Communist in Stalinist Russia.*

Made in the USA
Charleston, SC
08 November 2010